THE **BOOK** OF
OUTDOOR
GAMES

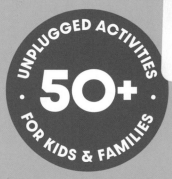

UNPLUGGED ACTIVITIES
· **50+** ·
FOR KIDS & FAMILIES

T0001120

BY EMILY PHILPOTT

CIDER MILL
PRESS

BOOK
PUBLISHERS

THE BOOK OF OUTDOOR GAMES

13-Digit ISBN: 978-1-64643-420-6
10-Digit ISBN: 1-64643-420-X

This book may be ordered by mail from the publisher. Please include $5.99 for postage and handling. Please support your local bookseller first!

Books published by Cider Mill Press Book Publishers are available at special discounts for bulk purchases in the United States by corporations, institutions, and other organizations. For more information, please contact the publisher.

Cider Mill Press Book Publishers
"Where good books are ready for press"
501 Nelson Place
Nashville, Tennessee 37214

cidermillpress.com

Printed in Malaysia

Typography: Dazzle Unicase, Poppins

All vectors used under official license from Shutterstock.com.

23 24 25 26 27 OFF 5 4 3 2 1
First Edition

CONTENTS

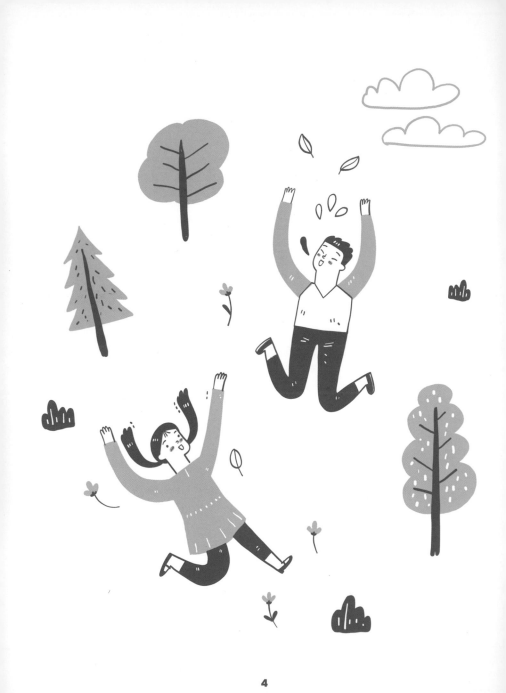

INTRODUCTION

All creatures love to play! Whether puppies or penguins or people—we all do things that have no explanation other than that they are "fun." While we all have the instincts to game and practice frivolity, it's easy to be caught on the spot without a specific activity in mind. This book is meant to serve as a tool to solve that problem. Inside, you'll find games that will help your group get to know one another, as well as games for when folks want to chill, run, cool off, or just be silly. Though many of these games could be adapted to be played inside, they're really intended to be played outside. Nothing quite compares to the magic of creating a challenge that incorporates the natural world, with no jungle gyms or screens required! Use this book as a jumping-off point to find games that work for your group and the adaptations that make them uniquely yours. Above all, remember to take breaks from daily routines and go outside to connect with your playful self—have fun!

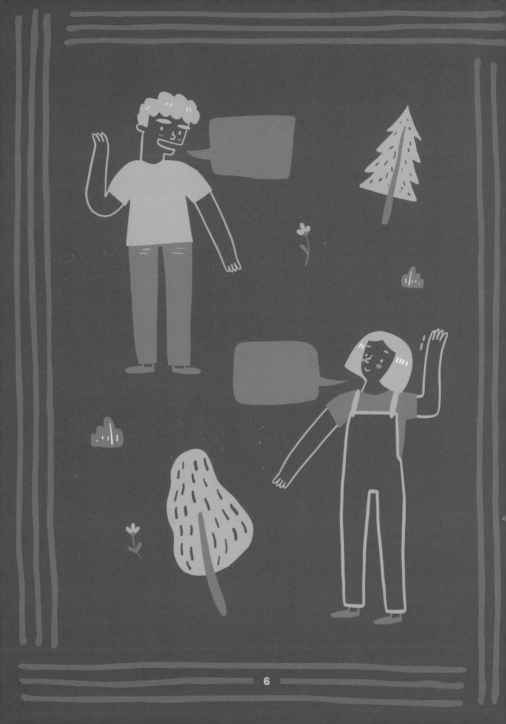

NAME GAMES AND ICEBREAKERS

1

ZOMBIE TAG

AGES – ANY
GROUP SIZE – 6 OR MORE
TIME – 15 MINUTES
MATERIALS – CONES

"Zombie Tag" is a fun way to get your group to practice learning each other's names. To set up, create a small boundary with the cones. For 12 people, a good starting point is a 10'x10' space.

Everyone should begin mingling within the boundary, moving at zombie speed. The creepier the walking, the better!

Choose one person to start the game as "it." They should look down while the rest of the group mingles about in the space, look up, and then start pursuing the first person they see. The "it" person should have their arms extended out in front of them like a zombie hungry for brains.

The target can only evade the zombie "it" person in two ways: walking away at zombie speed or calling out the name of another person in the group.

Once a name has been called, that person becomes the "it" zombie, targeting the first person they see.

If someone gets tagged, they move to the outside of the square, but not before selecting a new person to be "it."

The game continues until there are just two zombies remaining in the square. Tie break however you see fit, but probably not with a "brain-eating contest."

PRO TIP: Shrink the boundary as needed as the group of zombies dwindles. This keeps the game interesting and fast-paced, even though no one should be moving faster than a "walk."

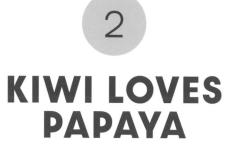

KIWI LOVES PAPAYA

AGES – ANY
GROUP SIZE – 6 OR MORE
TIME – 15 MINUTES
MATERIALS – CONES

For this fruit-lover's name game, start by forming a circle of cones. There should be a cone for everyone but one person in the circle. The extra person will start in the middle.

Have each person introduce themselves so that everyone can hear the names.

Game play flows by having one person "pass" the energy target by saying, "<u>My name loves someone else's name from the circle</u>." For example, I might say, "Emily loves Lindy," to pass the energy target. Lindy now has to say, "Lindy loves <u>someone else's name</u>," to pass the target again.

Meanwhile, the person in the middle of the circle is walking around and trying to tag the person with the energy target before they can express their undying love to someone else in the group.

If the person in the middle is able to tag someone, they switch spots with that individual and game play continues.

Endless variations of this game exist! Have each player come up with a fruit name that starts with the same letter as their first name (Amelia could be "apple," but Zoey might have a tougher time generating an alias). Is calling out getting too easy? Try having everyone create a unique dance move to represent themselves!

HERE I STAND

AGES – ANY
GROUP SIZE – 6 OR MORE
TIME – 15 MINUTES
MATERIALS – CONES

Woohoo! Another name game! To set this one up, create a circle of cones where each player has a cone and there is one extra cone.

The game begins with someone standing next to the empty cone. They should step and slide into the empty space, ideally with some Broadway-worthy flair. As they slide, they say, "Here I stand..."

Next, the person who is now across the empty space from them should slide into their old space, saying, "In the grass..."

Again, the person who newly finds themselves next to the empty space should slide over, saying,

"With my friend, _____" and fill in the blank with someone else in the circle.

The person whose name was called should run over to the empty cone, leaving their old cone behind and vacant.

Now, the people on either side of the empty cone will race to slide in and start the "Here I stand..." cascade.

The game continues on—try to get as fast as possible!

TARP DROP

AGES - ANY
GROUP SIZE - 6 OR MORE
TIME - 15 MINUTES
MATERIALS - A TARP OR BIG BLANKET

This name game tests both the memory of names as well as the ability to think quickly under pressure. To begin, divide the group into two teams. Two people will be needed to "host" the game.

Have the groups standing on either side of a tarp or blanket that is suspended vertically in the air. The tarp or blanket should be creating an opaque wall that blocks each team from seeing the other.

Each team should send a champion, quietly, up close to the tarp.

The hosts will then quickly lower the tarp. Now that the challengers can see each other, they are racing to call out the name of their opponent.

The slower challenger moves to the victorious side, and the hosts reset the tarp.

The game continues until there is one team to rule them all, or when everyone is all on one side of the tarp.

There are lots of fun variations of this game! One favorite is having the challengers face away from each other and then rely on the group to give hints about the identity of the opponent. Another is to have the whole group stand together with one person missing from each—the groups are racing to identify the missing person by name!

TRAIN WRECK

AGES – ANY
GROUP SIZE – 6 OR MORE
TIME – 15 MINUTES
MATERIALS – CONES

"Train Wreck" is a game that allows players to get to know a little more about one another. To set up, create a circle of cones with enough cones for all players but one. The remaining player starts in the middle of the circle.

The player in the middle begins the game by calling out, "Switch if you <u>have the same fun fact as me</u>." For example, they might say, "Switch if you have blue eyes."

At this point, everyone who has blue eyes should leave their spot to find a new spot. The person in the middle is also trying to find a spot at a cone.

Whoever does not find a new cone is now the person in the middle and should call out a new fun fact.

Play should continue this way, with the person in the middle calling out fun facts and folks switching spots accordingly.

Periodically, the person in the middle can call, "Train wreck!"—it may not surprise you to hear that this means everyone has to find a new cone. Be careful not to bump into anyone!

To enhance game play, players should not be allowed to go back to the same cone they started at or to a cone directly next to them. Kids can also be tempted to make fun facts that only target a specific player, and this should also be avoided.

BODYGUARD

AGES - ANY
GROUP SIZE - 6 OR MORE
TIME - 5 MINUTES
MATERIALS - NONE

"Bodyguard" is a good way to ease the tension of being with a new group and just get folks moving! To set up, all you need is a flat and open space.

Begin by having everyone silently select someone else in the group to be their bodyguard. Everyone should keep their selections a secret!

Similarly, everyone should also secretly identify someone in the group who is their assassin, but make sure the word doesn't get out!

Now, the objective is for everyone to keep their bodyguard in a direct line between them and their assassin. To do this, everyone should continuously move around the area in order to stay "safe."

After a minute or two, "freeze" the game and see how people did at keeping away from their assassins.

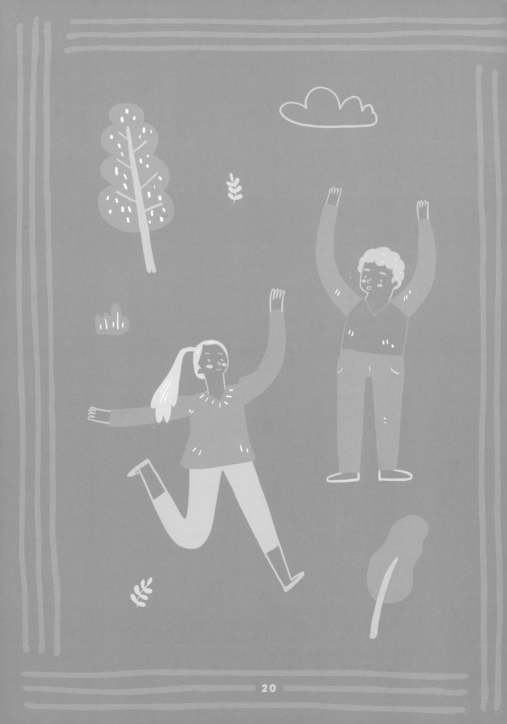

STATIONARY GAMES

ROCK, PAPER, SCISSORS, SPLITS!

AGES – ANY
GROUP SIZE – 2 OR MORE
TIME – 5 MINUTES
MATERIALS – NONE

"Rock, Paper, Scissors, Splits!" is a fun variation on the classic game we all use to settle silly debates. To play, have the challengers start with one foot forward, toe to toe. Each person's other foot should be behind their front foot, heel to toe.

Play "Rock, Paper, Scissors" as you have before— chant "rock, paper, scissors, shoot!" and each player should reveal a hand signal for their weapon of choice. A closed fist represents "rock," a flat palm represents "paper," and two fingers in a peace sign represents "scissors." Rock beats scissors, scissors beats paper, and paper beats rock.

Now, the twist comes in!

After each round, the losing opponent should slide their back foot one shoe length away, slowly creeping toward their legs being in a "split" position. The front feet of the opponents should stay touching, toe to toe.

The game continues until one person can no longer hold the "split" and surrenders. In light of this, it's probably wise to play on a grippy surface, but to each their own!

NINJA

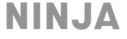

AGES – ANY
GROUP SIZE – 3 OR MORE
TIME – 15 MINUTES
MATERIALS – NONE

"Ninja" is a favorite among kids of all ages! To play, all you need is a flat and open space.

Begin by having everyone start with their feet touching in the middle of a circle.

Next, the leader should call, "NINJA!" and everyone should simultaneously jump out from the center of the circle, away from one another. Each person should freeze exactly as they landed—don't move the feet, body, or hands!

Now that everyone is spread out, the leader can begin play by making *one fluid movement* that can include one jump to try to touch their hand to someone else's hand. It's important to note that there cannot be multiple steps or multiple directions of arm movement.

The person being attacked can also make *one fluid movement* to evade the attack.

If the attacker makes contact with a hand (anywhere from the wrist down), the attackee "loses" that hand and must hold it behind their back.

Play continues around the circle clockwise. Ninjas should only be moving if they are the attacker or the one being attacked!

Ninjas are "out" when they lose both of their hands.

The winner is whoever is the last person standing!

To avoid folks being bored once out, you can start a second group of "Recreational Ninjas" who can continue playing while the "Super Bowl Ninjas" duke it out to determine the ultimate champion.

LOOK DOWN, LOOK UP

AGES – ANY
GROUP SIZE – 10 OR MORE
TIME – 10 MINUTES
MATERIALS – NONE

As the name suggests, "Look Down, Look Up" is a pretty simple game. To set up, have your group form a circle where everyone is facing inward.

The leader should call, "Look down!" and, you guessed it, everyone should look at their toes.

Next, the leader calls, "Look up!" at which point everyone should look at someone else in the circle, trying to make eye contact. Each person should be picking one person and looking directly at them—no wishy-washy stares!

If any two people are making eye contact, they should give a loud screech and run out of the circle. This game is also called "Screaming Toes" for this reason.

Once the first people have left, they should form a new circle and continue game play.

This repeats, and people should be moving back and forth from one circle to another.

The game can end whenever the giggles stop or after the group re-forms one big circle.

ZEN MASTER

AGES – ANY
GROUP SIZE – 2 OR MORE
TIME – 10 MINUTES
MATERIALS – A PEBBLE OR SMALL
OBJECT FOR EACH PLAYER

"Zen Master" is a fun and easy game that can be played anywhere with gravel, acorns, or similarly sized objects. To begin, have each player find their small object. It should be small enough that they can easily wrap their hand around it.

Next, each person should hold their hand out flat in front of them, palm facing down. Each person should place their small object on the back of their hand. It should be able to sit securely on the back of their hand if they are not moving.

The object of the game is to knock the object off of the back of the other players' hands, but each player has to make sure that they don't lose their own object! Everyone should be using balance and measured movements to succeed—players are not allowed to hold their object in any way.

The winner is the last person standing with their object still resting on their hand.

This is another game with endless variations! Players can rest the object on just the tip of one finger, or bend their arm so that the object can rest on an elbow. The game could also be set up as a tournament or as an all-out melee.

BOB THE WEASEL

AGES – ANY
GROUP SIZE – 8 OR MORE
TIME – 15 MINUTES
MATERIALS – ONE SMALL OBJECT
THAT CAN BE FULLY CONCEALED
BETWEEN TWO HANDS

"Bob the Weasel" is a fun game that encourages paying attention and being quiet—great for a moment when the group needs a cooldown!

To set up, have everyone sit in a circle with one person in the middle as the "Detective." The circle should be small enough that each player can comfortably reach those next to them with two hands closed together in front of them.

The object of the game is to continuously pass the small object throughout the circle. To do this, players should all cup their hands together in front of them, whether or not they have the object. Each player should gently shake their hands and mime as if they are passing and receiving the object—to an outsider, it should look like each person has an object they are passing. Encourage everyone to act their hearts out as they pretend to pass the object!

The Detective begins their role with their eyes closed, so that the object can be passed a few times and its location concealed. They should be standing in the middle—once they open their eyes, they are doing their best to identify Bob the Weasel, aka whoever has the object. Depending on the group's size and skill, a limit should be set on the number of guesses. Three guesses is typically a good starting point.

If the Detective identifies Bob the Weasel, Bob the Weasel becomes the new Detective and the game begins again.

FROGGY MURDER

AGES – ANY, BUT BEST FOR 12 AND UNDER
GROUP SIZE – 8 OR MORE
TIME – 10 MINUTES
MATERIALS – NONE

Despite its name, "Froggy Murder" is a pretty silly and lighthearted game. It's a favorite, especially among the younger crowd.

To set up, have the group form a seated circle where every person can clearly see one another. One person should remain out of the circle to serve as the "Detective."

While the Detective's eyes are closed, silently select someone to be the "Frog." Everyone else is a hapless little "Fly."

The Frog's objective is to eat all the Flies, without getting caught by the Detective. To do so, the

Frog must make eye contact with a Fly and subtly stick out their tongue. The Fly should then clutch their heart and "die" in a dramatic fashion. Each Fly is allowed to delay up to 3 seconds past their demise so as to deter suspicion.

Meanwhile, the Detective is standing in the middle of the circle, looking around to investigate the scene. The Detective is allowed three guesses to identify the Frog. The Detective should not stand and only face one direction—they must be consistently looking around.

If the Detective successfully identifies the Frog, or if the Frog successfully eats all the Flies without being caught, the Frog becomes the new Detective. Once a new Frog is chosen, the game begins again!

HONEY, IF YOU LOVE ME

AGES – ANY, BUT BEST FOR 12 AND UNDER
GROUP SIZE – 6 OR MORE
TIME – 10 MINUTES
MATERIALS – NONE

"Honey, If You Love Me" is the perfect game for the silly jokesters in your life. All you need is a group that's ready to put on a show!

To set up, have the group form a standing circle with one person in the middle. Leave plenty of room in the middle of the circle for shenanigans!

The players that are forming the circle should be doing their best to keep a straight face, regardless of the goofiness that happens in front of them.

The player in the middle of the circle is trapped there until they can get one of the others to crack a smile. In order to do so, they should approach another player face to face and say, "Honey, if you love me, would you please, please smile?" They should be encouraged to put their own spin on the phrase, or make funny faces, to add some flair.

If the person on the outside is able to listen without breaking a grin, their trial isn't quite over! As we know, one should never ignore a request from their "honey"!

To truly get out of the woods, the person in the circle must say, "Honey, I love you, but I just can't smile."

If they still do not smile, the middle person should continue their quest with a new victim and hope that next time their jokes do not fall flat.

Once they get a target to smile, the two switch places and roles and the game continues!

LITTLE SALLY WALKER

AGES – ANY
GROUP SIZE – 6 OR MORE
TIME – 10 MINUTES
MATERIALS – NONE

Similar to "Honey, If You Love Me," "Little Sally Walker" gives theatrical players a chance to perform and have a laugh.

To play, the group should form a circle with one person in the middle. That person is "Little Sally Walker" and should be skipping around the interior perimeter of the circle.

While they skip, everyone should sing the following: "Little Sally Walker, walking down the street, she didn't know what to do, so she stopped in front of me!"

At the end of that verse, Little Sally Walker should stop in front of another player and begin doing a dance of their choosing. While they dance, everyone is singing: "Hey girl, do your thing, do your thing, don't stop!" The person in front of them should be mimicking their moves.

At the end of this verse, the players switch spots and there's a new Sally Walker in town!

After the swap, there is another verse of "Hey girl, do your thing, do your thing, don't stop!" still doing the original dance move.

The game continues with the new Sally Walker skipping around to the original verse. Keep going until everyone has had a chance to be in the middle, or until folks have had their fill of performing.

ALPHABET CHALLENGE

AGES – ANY
GROUP SIZE – 2 OR MORE
TIME – 15 MINUTES
MATERIALS – NONE

Need to fill some time or re-collect your group? "Alphabet Challenge" could be the perfect choice!

To play, choose a category, such as "animals," "foods," "restaurants," or whatever your heart desires. The object of the game is to take turns naming an answer for each letter of the alphabet, in order.

Encourage players not to give hints unless asked, no matter how excited they are to have figured out an answer!

In my experience, even the kids who resist participating get sucked into the challenge for the chance to be the one to find a restaurant that begins with "X."

GROUP COUNT

AGES – ANY
GROUP SIZE – 5 OR MORE
TIME – 15 MINUTES
MATERIALS – NONE

"Group Count" is a good game for anyone interested in team building, especially with a focus on patience.

The object of the game is simple—all the group needs to do is count to 10! Where's the challenge? Well, no one in the group should speak at the same time as another. Any time more than one person speaks, the count resets to 0 and they must restart.

To add a degree of difficulty, you can instruct the group not to go in the order of their physical arrangement. Still too easy? Have the group keep their eyes closed the whole time or increase the count from 10 to a higher number.

17

POWER OF 10

AGES – ANY
GROUP SIZE – 5 OR MORE
TIME – 5 MINUTES
MATERIALS – NONE

Not to be confused with the "Group Count" challenge, "Power of 10" is a strategy game for the mathematically inclined.

To play, have the group sit or stand in a circle. The object of the game is for the group to count to 10, but whichever individual says "ten" is eliminated.

On their turn, each player can increase the count by either 1 or 2. For example, the first player might say "one," the second player could say "two" or "two, three," and so on.

Play continues until all players but one have been eliminated. Games conclude quickly, but feel free to play as many rounds as you can count!

21

AGES - ANY
GROUP SIZE - 5 OR MORE
TIME - 15 MINUTES
MATERIALS - ONE SMALL OBJECT
THAT CAN BE FULLY CONCEALED
BETWEEN TWO HANDS

"21" is another numbers game, but this time with more emphasis on patterns. To play, have the group sit or stand in a circle. Each player takes a turn as the group counts up to 21, adding one number in sequence at a time.

Each time someone reaches "twenty-one," they can add a rule to any number that has not yet been altered. Examples of rules include "instead of saying 'two,' clap three times," or "instead of saying 'fifteen,' say 'fourteen' again." Players are invited to be as creative or tricky as possible!

After a new rule is added, the group starts over at "one" and works to count up to 21, making sure to remember all the added rules.

If a player makes a mistake and forgets a rule, the count restarts at "one."

Play as long as the group can focus, or until there is a rule for every number and the group can successfully do the new count. Good luck!

GROUP JUGGLE

AGES – ANY
GROUP SIZE – 8 OR MORE
TIME – 15 MINUTES
MATERIALS – SEVERAL TOSSABLE
OBJECTS, ENOUGH FOR EVERY
PLAYER IN THE GROUP

"Group Juggle" gives folks a chance to throw things, but with enough boundaries that things don't get too out of hand.

To play, have the group stand in a circle. Start off by tossing a single object to someone else in the circle. Each player should continue to toss the object on, making sure not to throw it to someone next to them or to someone who has already received the object. Make sure each person remembers whom they threw to, and who threw it to them!

Once the last player receives the object, they should throw it back to the person who initiated the sequence.

Next, toss the single object around in the same sequence to practice. If successful, add in another object to be tossed following the same sequence.

After each successful round, add in another object. Challenge your group to be able to reach one object per person.

If things are getting too easy, have the group shuffle about to new locations, but keep the same tossing sequence. Can your group handle the juggle?

DRUM MAJOR

AGES – ANY
GROUP SIZE – 6 OR MORE
TIME – 15 MINUTES
MATERIALS – NONE

"Drum Major" encourages creativity and focus, all with an air of intrigue. To set up, have the group sit or stand in a circle, with one person in the middle as the "Detective."

While the Detective's eyes are closed, silently select another player to be the "Drum Major."

The Drum Major is responsible for making the beat, all while avoiding the suspicion of the Detective. To do so, they should be creating percussion patterns by patting their laps or clapping or snapping. All other players should be casually watching and following the Drum Major, but they should not be drawing suspicion! Good band-mates should support their leader, after all.

Meanwhile, the Detective is standing in the middle of the circle, trying to identify the Drum Major within three guesses.

If they successfully identify the Drum Major, or run out of guesses, the game is over. Invite the Drum Major to be the new Detective, silently select a new Drum Major, and let the game continue.

To add to the air of mystery, you can select the Drum Major as a complete secret from everyone.

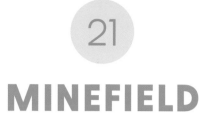

MINEFIELD

AGES – ANY
GROUP SIZE – 5 OR MORE
TIME – 15 MINUTES
MATERIALS – 25 POLY SPOTS,
CONES, OR OTHER WAY TO CREATE
A 5X5 GRID OF PLACES

"Minefield" is both a memory challenge and a team-building challenge. To set up, create a 5x5 grid of spaces that the players can stand on. Additionally, you should make a predetermined "route" through your grid. To make sure you don't forget, it's probably best to write it down.

The object of the game for the players is to navigate through the minefield to get to the other side. In order to do so, they can only move one space at a time, one person at a time.

If a player steps on a space that is "off route," simply shake your head "no" at them. They should then return to the start. Now the next person gets a chance.

If a player steps on a "safe" spot, nod your head "yes." The player can then make another move, either forward, backward, or to the side. The player can continue to make moves until they make a mistake.

All the players on the sideline should be paying attention! On their turn, they should be continuing to try to find the safe route, based on the information discovered by those before them.

After a player crosses fully to safety, it is up to each of the remaining players to make the same journey, following the same path.

For an added challenge, you can instruct players not to talk to each other or give hints.

To extend play, you can make as many "routes" as you'd like, or you can have blank grids on which players can make their own route.

ULTIMATE CHAMPION

AGES – ANY
GROUP SIZE – 6 OR MORE
TIME – 5–10 MINUTES
MATERIALS – A SMALL WHITEBOARD
OR SIMILAR WRITING SURFACE

Forget Fantasy Football—"Ultimate Champion" is a game that allows players to play out the tournament of their dreams.

To play, ask each player to think of the individual, either real or fictitious, that they think could defeat all others. Think John Cena or Boss Baby or Dua Lipa—or anyone else that could take out the competition.

Once each player has determined their fighter, draw out a tournament bracket and fill it in with the challengers.

For each match, the players get a chance to give a one-minute elevator pitch of why their fighter would win. After both players have their chance to speak, the other players get to vote on the winner.

The winner of each round proceeds to the next level of the tournament, until one player defeats all others to become...the ULTIMATE CHAMPION!

CELEBRITIES

AGES - 12 OR OLDER
GROUP SIZE - 6 OR MORE
TIME - 15 MINUTES
MATERIALS - SCRAP PAPER AND ENOUGH
WRITING UTENSILS FOR EVERYONE

"Celebrities" is a favorite for rainy days when stuck under a tarp or in a park shelter.

To play, give each player a small piece of paper and a pen or pencil.

Instruct everyone to write down the name of someone everyone would know. This could be someone famous on a world stage, or famous among your group.

Once everyone has written down a name, collect each piece of paper. Read through every name twice, but no more. Everyone should pay attention—remembering the names is half the challenge!

When it is their turn, each player should try to guess who wrote down what name. If an individual guesses correctly, the freshly identified celebrity moves to join their team and, together, they can guess again.

If a player guesses incorrectly, their turn ends and the game moves on to the next person.

Play continues until one person guesses the identity of each player/celebrity.

Once half of the players have been identified, you can read through the celebrities again as a refresher if it seems needed. Part of the fun is remembering, or being strategically forgotten, after all!

ROCK BOCCE

AGES – ANY
GROUP SIZE – 2 OR MORE
TIME – 5 MINUTES
MATERIALS – 7 ROCKS OR SIMILAR
OBJECTS. MAKE SURE ONE OF THE ROCKS
IS DISTINCT FROM ALL THE REST!

There's always something magical about taking a favorite game and converting it to a more "rustic" version.

To play, first establish the boundaries for your throwing field, and establish the location from which all throws should begin. Feel free to create a field with obstacles such as trees or uneven terrain!

One player should throw the key rock out onto the playing field. This is now the target for all other throws.

Players take turns throwing rocks, trying to get as close to the target rock as possible. Three rocks per player is a good amount.

Whoever gets their rock closest to the target wins and gets to throw the next target for setup.

Be creative! Rather than tossing a target rock, use an existing boulder or tree as the target. Try different starting points for your throws!

The game can be extended on the front end by making a challenge out of players finding the coolest target rock, or finding the most interesting playing field.

YEE HAW

AGES – ANY
GROUP SIZE – 6 OR MORE
TIME – 15 MINUTES
MATERIALS – NONE

"Yee Haw" is all about connecting to some down-home roots, and spreading that to the rest of the group.

To play, have the group form a standing circle with a comfortable amount of space between each player.

The point of the game is to pass the "yee haw" energy around the circle, but there are specific ways to keep the energy flowing.

To pass the energy directly to the person on either side of you, make a closed fist and swing your arm, with your elbow at 90 degrees, in front of you and say, "Yee haw!" If a player uses their right arm to swing to the left, the energy passes to the left.

If a player uses their left arm to swing to the right, the energy passes to the right.

Whoever has the energy now can continue with the "yee haw" arm swing, or they can try a different method to pass.

The energy can be passed across the circle by a player stepping forward with their hands at their hips, as if their thumbs are looped through a belt loop, and pointing their finger at someone opposite them while saying, "Get down, lil dogie." The person who was pointed at receives the energy and passes it on to someone else, using "yee haw" or "get down, lil dogie."

If your group gets the hang of these rules, here are some more you can add, or you can make up your own!

"Ba ting!" In response to "get down, lil dogie," use your belt buckle to deflect the "get down, lil dogie" to someone else!

"Hay barn!" In response to "yee haw," put your hands over your head to make a roof—the "yee haw" goes over your head and to the next person in line.

"Herd on the loose!" Everyone has to find a new spot in the circle. Whoever made the call makes a new call once they reach their new spot.

TRIVIA SPLASH

AGES – ANY
GROUP SIZE – 6 OR MORE
TIME – 15 MINUTES
MATERIALS – A WATER BOTTLE, A BUCKET
(OR ANY OTHER VESSEL THAT CAN HOLD
SOME WATER), AND PLENTY OF WATER!

Need to cool off in the middle of a hot summer day? Take a break from the heat and the running around with "Trivia Splash."

To play, have the group form a circle with you in the middle. You'll need your bucket handy and filled with water, with plenty of water on hand to replenish it.

The game is simple—ask the players a trivia question, and if they get it wrong (or right—you can decide), they get a splash from the bucket.

This game is a fun way to review concepts that you have been learning about during your time together, or a silly way to get to know each other. It often seems that the sillier the question, the better!

Keep playing until everyone has cooled off and had their fill.

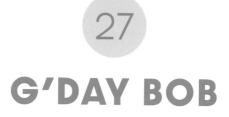

G'DAY BOB

AGES – ANY, THOUGH OLDER KIDS MAY HAVE AN EASIER TIME

GROUP SIZE – 4 OR MORE

TIME – 15 MINUTES

MATERIALS – NONE

If you're looking for a tongue twister, look no further than "G'day Bob." All that you need to play is to have the group sit in a circle and enough patience to try to play.

This is a word game where the speaking is passed around the circle. The lines go like this:

Player 1 to Player 2: "G'day Bob"

P2 to P1: "G'day Bob"

P1 to P2: "Say 'G'day' to Bob, Bob"

P2 to P3: "G'day Bob"

Repeat around the circle.

If someone makes a mistake, their new name is "Sheila," and everyone must remember to alter the statement when referring to them, lest they also become "Sheila."

For example:

P2 to P3: "G'day Sheila"

P3 to P2: "G'day Bob"

P2 to P3: "Say g'day to Bob, Sheila"

If a Sheila makes a mistake, they can now only say "wallaby" in a singsong voice.

The last person to remain "Bob" wins the game!

SPLAT!

AGES - ANY
GROUP SIZE - 6 OR MORE
TIME - 15 MINUTES
MATERIALS - NONE

"Splat!" is a good way to practice paying attention under the guise of simply trying to be the last one standing. To set up, have your group form a circle with one person in the middle.

The person in the middle points at someone in the circle and says, "Splat!" This person now should crouch down.

Next, the people on either side of the crouching person are racing to point at each other and say "splat!" Whoever is the slowest is out. If they say it at the exact same time, they can both stay in.

Keep playing until you are down to two players. You can break the tie however you please (although there is a great tiebreaking strategy for this game on page 125).

The winner can be the next person to play in the center of the circle!

Be sure to emphasize that the person in the center should be very clear about whom they are pointing to—instruct them to point both with their body and with their hand to reduce confusion.

Another way to play this is to determine "outs" by catching those who break the rules—for instance, if a player were to call "splat" when they weren't supposed to, if a player didn't crouch when pointed to, if they waited too long to say "splat," etc. When your group gets too quick for the first version, this variation can be a good way to keep them on their toes!

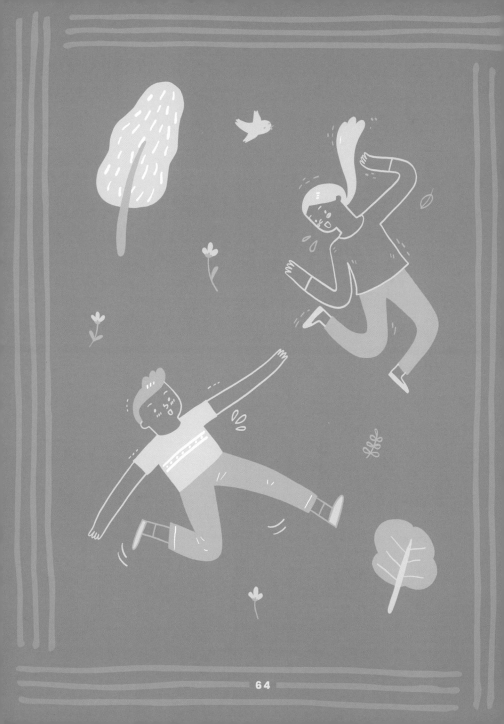

MOVING GAMES

FASTEST TAG IN THE WEST

AGES – ANY
GROUP SIZE – 6 OR MORE
TIME – 15 MINUTES
MATERIALS – NONE

This is a long-standing favorite game among players of all ages, due to the way it elevates the energy of tag with a new level of strategy.

In "Fastest Tag in the West," everyone is "it." You read that right—this game *does* have a healthy dose of chaos!

To set up, first establish the boundaries of your playing field.

Every player should be running around the playing field, but trying not to let anyone get too close.

The object is to be the last player standing and to "tag" as many people as possible by gently touching them. Be sure that your target doesn't turn around and tag you first!

Once someone gets tagged, they crouch down into a squat, but their chances of winning are not totally gone! They should keep an eye on the person who tagged them as they crouch. Once their tagger gets tagged, they are back in the game!

If two people tag each other at the same time, they should play "Rock, Paper, Scissors" to settle the tie. The loser got "tagged" and the winner goes on to try to tag more targets.

This game goes on until there is only one person standing, or until folks need a water break. As the host of the game, you may choose to call a "jail break" if the game seems to be stagnating.

A fun variant that stays popular is to make the game "adults vs. children"—kids love to band together to try to take out the grown-ups!

TOILET TAG

AGES - ANY
GROUP SIZE - 6 OR MORE
TIME - 15 MINUTES
MATERIALS - NONE

It's hard to deny that any game with the word "toilet" in its name will get kids excited. Get some energy and giggles out with a round or two of "Toilet Tag"!

To play, set up the boundaries of your playing field.

This game follows the general premise of tag—one person is "it," and they are trying to tag all the others.

When someone gets tagged, they should drop down to one knee and put their hand out like a toilet flusher.

They can be saved by another player if they choose to stop to "relieve themselves" by sitting down on the toilet seat formed by someone's knee and flushing the toilet using the hand "flusher."

You can even the odds by having multiple players be "it" or by switching up the "it" person periodically.

Have fun, and try not to get "flushed away"!

31

ELBOW TAG

AGES - ANY
GROUP SIZE - 8 OR MORE
TIME - 15 MINUTES
MATERIALS - NONE

Another variation of regular tag, "Elbow Tag" gives players a chance to run and play with built-in breaks.

To play, set up some boundaries on your playing field. Next, have everyone link arms with a partner.

Break up two partners. One should be "it," and the other should be the runner. If the "it" person tags the runner, the two players switch roles.

If the runner needs a break, they can link arms to one of the other pairs. When they do this, the person on the opposite side of them is now "bumped out" and is running from the "it" person.

The game keeps going until folks need a break that lasts a little longer than the reprieve of joining one of the elbow pairs!

32

BLOB TAG

AGES – ANY
GROUP SIZE – 8 OR MORE
TIME – 15 MINUTES
MATERIALS – NONE

Here is one final variation of tag (though it stands to reason that you could think of a million different versions on your own). "Blob Tag" adds a silly team aspect to the fray.

Set up by establishing play boundaries and choosing one person to be "it."

Whenever the "it" person tags someone, they link arms to form a blob. The newly formed blob now runs around and aims to tag more people to absorb them into the blob.

Game play continues until each player is part of the blob!

After a round, set up to play again! After all, it feels good to be part of something.

RED LIGHT, GREEN LIGHT

AGES – ANY
GROUP SIZE – 6 OR MORE
TIME – 10 MINUTES
MATERIALS – NONE

"Red Light, Green Light" is the quintessential instruction-following game—a great way to refocus your group while still getting some wiggles out.

To set up, establish a starting line and have all the players stand along it. You should go to the opposite end of the playing field to serve as the "stoplight."

Players are trying to cross the finish line where you stand, but they are only allowed to move when the conditions are right!

If you call "green light," players can run toward the finish, until they hear you call "red light." If anyone is moving still once you say "red light," they are sent back to the start!

Similarly, if you call "yellow light," players can walk toward the finish until you call "red light." Again, if they are moving after the "red light," or moving faster than a walk, they are sent back to the beginning.

The first player to cross the finish line wins!

Endless variants exist—try having the players move like animals or skip, or give others the chance to be the "stoplight" and call out instructions.

WHO STOLE MY WATER BOTTLE?

AGES – ANY
GROUP SIZE – 6 OR MORE
TIME – 15 MINUTES
MATERIALS – A WATER BOTTLE OR
OTHER SIMILAR OBJECT

"Who Stole My Water Bottle?" is reminiscent of "Red Light, Green Light." To play, have everyone line up on one end of a playing field. You should be on the opposite end, with your back to the others and the water bottle on the ground at your heels.

You are the water bottle "Guard." As Guard, you are trying to prevent the others from stealing your water bottle.

The others are only able to move while you are saying, "Who stole my water bottle?" Once you finish the line, you are able to turn around and face the group. If you see someone moving, you can send them back to the beginning of the field.

The challenge doesn't end once the players reach the bottle—they still have to get it back to the starting point while flying under the radar.

They are still only allowed to move while you are saying, "Who stole my water bottle?" Like before, you are able to send people back to the start if you see them moving. Additionally, you are able to make one guess each time as to who is holding the water bottle. If you are correct, the water bottle returns to its spot at your heels, and the group goes back to the starting line to try again.

The group is allowed to pass the water bottle among them while they move. They should also all try to be sneaky and hold a fake water bottle to try to throw you off the scent.

Keep playing as long as you want. Give the players a chance to be the Guard to keep things interesting!

GIVE ME BACK MY DUCKS

AGES – ANY
GROUP SIZE – 8 OR MORE
TIME – 15 MINUTES
MATERIALS – 2 HULA HOOPS, 6 RUBBER DUCKS (OR RUBBER CHICKENS, OR OTHER SILLY OBJECTS), AND CONES OR ROPE

"Give Me Back My Ducks" gives players the chance to run and work as a team, and the chance to yell out a silly battle cry!

To set up, establish the boundaries of the playing field. Next, use your cones or rope to divide the boundary in half. On each half, place a hula hoop on the ground and place three rubber ducks in each hoop. Divide your players into two teams.

The game begins with a rousing yell of "Give me back my ducks!"

The object of the game for each team is to collect all the ducks into their team's hula hoop. To do so, players must cross the borderline and try to grab a duck from the hula hoop and sneak it back.

Once a player crosses the borderline into enemy territory, they are at risk of getting tagged. If they get tagged, they are sent to "jail," where they must wait for a teammate to tag them out or for you to call a "jail break." If they make it to the hula hoop, they are safe while they stand inside, but are vulnerable again once they step out to try to run back "home," so they had better make it quick!

All ducks are always in play, so the game can continue for quite a while. You can adjust the number of ducks to suit your group—fewer or more as needed.

Be sure to offer some "time-outs" for players to drink water and rest!

SPUD

AGES - ANY
GROUP SIZE - 6 OR MORE
TIME - 15 MINUTES
MATERIALS - A KICKBALL OR
SIMILAR OBJECT

"Spud" combines the game of "HORSE" with dodgeball.

To begin, assign each player, including you, a number, increasing from "one." Players should remember their number for the rest of the game.

Next, have all players form a tight circle around you while you are holding the ball. Throw the ball straight up in the air, as high as you can, and call out the number of another player in the group. Make sure not to call your own number!

While the ball is in the air, everyone, including you, should run out radially from the center to get as far away as possible.

Meanwhile, the person whose number got called should be trying to grab the ball, rather than running away. Once they catch the ball, they should yell, "SPUD!"

When everyone hears "SPUD!" they should freeze where they stand.

The person with the ball is now allowed two steps closer to any player. Once they take their steps, they can roll or throw the ball to try to hit another player.

Players in the field are not allowed to move their feet from where they stopped after "SPUD!" was called, but they can move at the knee or torso to try to dodge the ball.

If a player gets hit by the ball, they get an "S," or, if they already have an "S," they get a "P." Conversely, if the thrower misses the target, they get the letter added onto their tally.

Whoever was targeted by the throw is now the person to start the sequence—everyone should gather back in the middle around them while they throw the ball into the air and call out a new number.

The game ends when someone has all the letters of "SPUD."

WHAT TIME IS IT, MR. FOX?

AGES – ANY
GROUP SIZE – 4 OR MORE
TIME – 10 MINUTES
MATERIALS – NONE

To play "What Time Is It, Mr. Fox?" all you need is to set up a starting line and then stand somewhere opposite.

All the players should stand along the starting line. They should collectively call out, "What time is it, Mr. Fox?"

You are "Mr. Fox" and should respond, "__ o'clock!" —whatever time you say is the number of steps everyone has to take toward you. For example, if you answer "10 o'clock," players must take 10 steps closer to you. The steps can be however big or small the players choose.

After each round, the players call out again, "What time is it, Mr. Fox?" until, eventually, you answer, "MIDNIGHT!"

Once you call "MIDNIGHT!" it is a race back to the starting line, with you chasing the players back, trying to tag someone before they cross. Whoever you tag is the new "Mr. Fox," and the game begins again!

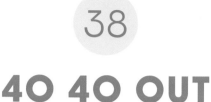

40 40 OUT

AGES - ANY
GROUP SIZE - 5 OR MORE
TIME - 15 MINUTES
MATERIALS - NONE

"40 40 Out" is a helpful tool for learning the names of your group while still having the chance to run around.

To play, set up a "base" tree, or similar object. One person is "it," and the rest should go hide in the playing field.

The "it" person starts at the base tree and then goes in search of hidden players. As soon as they spot someone, they should race back to the base and try to call, "40 40 _____ out," filling the player's name in the blank. Meanwhile, the person they spotted is also trying to race back to the base, where they would call, "40 40 _____ in," filling in the blank with their own name.

If the "it" person wins the race, the other player is out. If the player wins the race, they remain in play to try another round.

The game continues until everyone has been found. You can play more rounds with the people who stayed "in," or, choose a new "it" person from that pool and start the game again.

50-YARD SCREAM

AGES – ANY
GROUP SIZE – 1 OR MORE
TIME – 3 MINUTES
MATERIALS – NONE

This game really is just a chance for anyone and everyone to release some frustration or other loud energy.

Have everyone line up on a starting line, ideally on one end of a wide-open space. When you call "go," everyone should take a deep breath and run as far as they can across the field. What's the catch? Everyone should be yelling as loud as they can! Once people lose their breath, they have to stop wherever the scream ends. The winner is whoever makes it the farthest across the field before their scream runs out.

Go forth and release!

40

SLACKJAW

AGES – ANY
GROUP SIZE – 2 OR MORE
TIME – 10 MINUTES
MATERIALS – NONE

The object of "Slackjaw" is to get your opponent to smile while maintaining a straight face of your own.

Players choose an opponent and face them on the field. The weapon of choice? A silly dance! Players should pull out their wackiest moves to get their opponent to smile. Additionally, each player should "glue" their elbows to their sides—no flailing! The first person to smile loses.

You can play tournament style, with a bracket, or follow a structure similar to "Biggest Fan" (see page 88) and have the losers become cheerleaders until an ultimate champion is found. Add to the atmosphere by playing music.

BIGGEST FAN

AGES – ANY
GROUP SIZE – 8 OR MORE, BUT
THE BIGGER THE BETTER!
TIME – 5 MINUTES
MATERIALS – NONE

"Biggest Fan" is another take on the classic "Rock, Paper, Scissors," but with the added element of crazed fandom.

To play, everyone should select one opponent to challenge in a single, sudden-death round of "Rock, Paper, Scissors."

The winner moves on to find another opponent, while the loser becomes their "biggest fan," cheering them on with the kind of madness the world expects during the World Cup or, more locally, the Super Bowl.

Each time a player wins, they absorb their opponent and entourage into their fan base, until one player has reached the echelon of A-list celebrities or the person who brings Doritos to the party, and everyone is cheering for them alone.

42

SHIPS AND SAILORS

AGES – ANY
GROUP SIZE – 6 OR MORE
TIME – 15 MINUTES
MATERIALS – NONE

"Ships and Sailors" follows the structure of "Simon Says," but with more aerobic activity involved.

When you call a command, the players must follow. If they make a mistake, they are out. Here are some possible commands:

"Ships" All players run to the left.

"Sailors" All players run to the right.

"Hit the Deck" Players drop to the ground and lie flat.

"Starfish" Players jump with their arms and legs out to form a star shape.

"Seasick" Players run backward and mime throwing up.

"Mermaid on a Rock" Players find a partner. One partner drops to one knee, and the other sits on their knee and twirls their hair.

"Three Sailors Rowing" Players form a group of three, stand in a line, and mime rowing a boat.

"Dinnertime" Players form a group of four, arrange in a circle facing in, and mime eating.

"Captain's Coming" Players freeze and put their hand over their eyes as a salute. Players should not move. If any commands are called, they should not be followed until you call, "At Ease." If anyone moves before then, they are out.

"At Ease" The Captain has left the area, and players can go back to following the commands as usual.

The game flows by you calling commands and players being eliminated until one person remains. Beware of unbreakable ties—sometimes the best competitors can't be shaken. As a last resort, you can yell, "Anchor!" and have your finalists each stand on one leg until only one remains.

43

FOUR CORNERS

AGES – ANY
GROUP SIZE – 5 OR MORE
TIME – 10 MINUTES
MATERIALS – NONE

Sometimes, it truly can be as simple as it sounds. To play "Four Corners," all you need is to set up four spots and identify them as "one," "two," "three," and "four."

You start in the middle of the rectangle, close your eyes, and count loudly to "ten."

Meanwhile, all the other players should be sneaking around and then choosing a corner to stay in. They should make sure to be in a corner before you finish counting to 10!

With your eyes still closed, call out the number of a corner. Anyone hiding in that corner is now "out."

This repeats until you get everyone out, or there is one person left. Once you get down to two or three players, you can shrink the playing field to just two of the corners.

The winner is now the new person in the center, and the game can begin again!

GIANTS, WIZARDS, TROLLS

AGES – ANY
GROUP SIZE – 6 OR MORE
TIME – 10 MINUTES
MATERIALS – ROPE OR CONES

"Giants, Wizards, Trolls" is another spin on "Rock, Paper, Scissors," but with a silly, fantasy twist.

First, divide the players into two teams. Each team should have a home base line, marked with cones. In between the two base lines, there should be rope or cones on the ground marking the meeting spot.

Giants present by each person in the group making themselves as big as possible, with their hands over their heads, posing as if ready to grab. Giants beat Trolls by stomping on them.

Wizards present by each person in the group extending a hand straight out as if holding a wand. Wizards beat Giants by casting a spell on them.

Trolls present by each person in the group crouching down low and bringing their hands together and wiggling their fingers. Trolls beat Wizards by tugging their beards.

Before each round, the players have 10 seconds to consult with their teammates and choose which pose to play.

At the end of the 10 seconds, all players should approach the middle line and be facing one another. On the count of three, each team should go to the pose they decided on. All players from a team should be in the same pose.

The losing team should then run back to their base line while the winning team chases them, trying to tag as many people as they can. Anyone who gets tagged goes to the other team.

The game continues until everyone is on the same team. Good luck!

45

CAMOUFLAGE

AGES - ANY
GROUP SIZE - 5 OR MORE
TIME - 15 MINUTES
MATERIALS - NONE

Is "Hide-and-Seek" too simple? Try "Camouflage" to add in a level of strategy!

To play, everyone starts in the middle of a playing field. The arena should include trees or other things that players can hide behind.

All players start in the middle, and one person should be chosen to be "it."

The "it" person should slowly and loudly count to "ten."

Meanwhile, all other players should hurry to find a hiding spot where they can't be seen from the "it" person's vantage.

At the end of the count, the "it" person can open their eyes and look around. They must stay in the same spot, but they can pivot in place and crouch down. If they see someone, they should call out a distinct descriptor and where they are hiding. For example, one might call, "Red T-shirt behind the willow oak"—if someone is wearing a red T-shirt in that hiding spot, they are out.

After the "it" person thinks they have found as many people as possible, they can take a single step in one direction and try again.

At this point, once they have found as many people as possible, the "it" person should close their eyes and count aloud to "ten" again. All remaining players must find a new hiding spot that is closer to the "it" person.

The "it" person follows the same search procedure as before.

For the final round, the "it" person closes their eyes, while the remaining players try to silently approach the "it" person to tag them. If the "it" person hears someone and points at them, that person is out. The first person to tag the "it" person wins the game and is the next "it" person for another round.

SARDINES

AGES – ANY
GROUP SIZE – 5 OR MORE
TIME – 15 MINUTES
MATERIALS – NONE

"Sardines" is another take on "Hide-and-Seek"; however, in this game, the "it" person starts out as the only one able to hide.

While the "it" person goes to hide, the other players count to 20. Once they reach the end of their count, players should fan out in search of the "it" person.

When someone finds the "it" person, instead of calling out the hiding spot, they should quietly join them in hiding, trying to squish into the spot like sardines in a can.

The game continues on while the players keep searching. Any time someone finds the hiding spot, they must join in, filling the sardine can tighter and tighter.

When the final player finds the group, the game ends. You can reset and have the final player become the new "it" person for the next round!

ROPEY STUMPY

AGES – 10 OR OLDER
GROUP SIZE – 2 OR MORE
TIME – 10 MINUTES
MATERIALS – A LONG LENGTH OF ROPE
AND TWO STABLE OBJECTS TO STAND ON
(SUCH AS MILK CRATES OR STUMPS)

"Ropey Stumpy" requires balance, strategy, and focus. To set up, place the two standing objects roughly 10 feet apart. The rope should be pooled in the middle of the objects, with one end reaching to either one.

Have a competitor stand on each object. Milk crates work well because they are stable and easy to stand on. Each competitor begins with one end of the rope in their hand.

When you call "go," players can begin to start pulling the rope through, to try to get to the middle of the rope. Once there is tension on the rope, players can tug the rope and release slack strategically, trying to get their opponent to step off their platform.

The winner is the last person standing on their platform. It sounds simple, but it's kind of tricky to find the best strategy and not lose balance! Good luck!

SECURITY GUARD

AGES – ANY
GROUP SIZE – 5 OR MORE
TIME – 10 MINUTES
MATERIALS – FLASHLIGHTS (OPTIONAL)

"Security Guard" is especially fun if played at night with flashlights! It's a great "back-pocket" game, even more so during the winter when days are short.

To play, choose one person to be "it" and give them the flashlight. Set the boundaries around your playing field.

The "it" person is a museum "Security Guard," and the rest of the players are statues that come alive at night. Any time the Security Guard is not look-ing, the statues are living large! They should be dancing and mingling and having a good time. However, if the Security Guard "catches" them by shining a flashlight on them and seeing them move, they are out. To stay in, statues should freeze in a statuesque pose any time they think the Security Guard is about to catch them.

The game continues until one statue is left—they become the Security Guard for the next round!

GHOST IN THE GRAVEYARD

AGES – ANY
GROUP SIZE – 5 OR MORE
TIME – 10 MINUTES
MATERIALS – FLASHLIGHTS (OPTIONAL)

Here's another good nighttime game for when daylight saving time shrinks program hours.

For setup, you should establish the boundaries and a tree or other location to serve as a "base."

One person is chosen to be the "Ghost," and they are given 20 seconds to find a hiding spot. All remaining players may now use their flashlights to go searching for the Ghost.

The first person to find the Ghost should yell, "Ghost in the graveyard!" to alert the others, as the Ghost is now trying to race them back to base and tag them on the way.

Whoever is tagged first is the next Ghost, and the game continues!

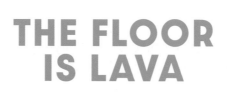

THE FLOOR IS LAVA

AGES – ANY
GROUP SIZE – 1 OR MORE
TIME – 15 MINUTES
MATERIALS – POLY SPOTS, POOL NOODLES, MILK CRATES, OR OTHER OBJECTS TO STAND ON

It's surely been a fantasy, or nightmare, of everyone's at some point—crossing a lava field by hopping from rock to rock to stay safe. Take a chance to live the dream by creating a precarious path from point A to point B, using any objects you can find that are stable enough to stand on—but don't make it too easy!

This game can be set up as an individual challenge—who can make it across the lava field with the least number of mistakes? Or, it can be set up as a team challenge—no one wins until everyone makes it across, and players should help each other through!

After each round, you can reset the course by rearranging the objects or taking objects away. Invite other players to help form the course or play solo—the choice is yours!

SHARKS AND MINNOWS

AGES – ANY
GROUP SIZE – 5 OR MORE
TIME – 15 MINUTES
MATERIALS – NONE

Shark Week can happen any time of year!

To set up for "Sharks and Minnows," create a playing field with safe zones marked on either end, and choose one person to be the "Shark."

All remaining players are "Minnows" and should gather in one of the safe zones.

Meanwhile, the Shark is in the middle of the field. When they are ready, they should look at the Minnows and call, "Come Minnows, come!" At this point, all the Minnows should run as fast as they can to the safe zone on the other side, while the shark tries to tag as many Minnows as possible.

A couple of versions exist here. Tagged Minnows can become "Anemones" and are frozen in place where they are tagged; they cannot move their feet, but they can bend and reach and try to tag Minnows when they run by. Alternatively, tagged Minnows can become Sharks and run freely to help tag Minnows.

After each running round, the Shark faces the Minnows and calls, "Come Minnows, come!"—the Minnows should be running from one side to the other, trying to escape being tagged.

The winner of the game is the last Minnow standing—they can become the next Shark!

52

RAINBOW SCAVENGER HUNT

AGES – ANY
GROUP SIZE – 1 OR MORE
TIME – 10 MINUTES
MATERIALS – NONE

This game is a great way to allow some movement, exploration, and calming energy.

The challenge is simple: each player should try to find something in nature for each rainbow color.

This game can be played solo or with multiple players, individually or in teams.

If you'd like there to be a winner, that can be the first person to complete the rainbow.

One of the best parts of this activity is having a "show-and-tell" at the end, allowing each player to display their treasures and ask questions about their origin.

Bonus points for the most unique finds!

53

BUCKET RACE

AGES – ANY
GROUP SIZE – 6 OR MORE
TIME – 15 MINUTES
MATERIALS – BUCKETS, CUPS, AND WATER

It is possible to run and play and still stay cool in the summer—games like "Bucket Race" make it so.

Players should be divided into two teams that stand in single-file lines.

To play, place a bucket full of water in front of each lined-up team. At the end of each team's line should be an empty bucket.

Give the player in the front of each line a cup. They can use the cup to scoop water from the bucket, and then they pass the cup full of water over their head to the person behind them, who does the same, until the last player is reached.

The last player in the line holds the cup over their head and tries to pour it into the empty bucket behind them.

To get the cup back to the front, players should reach between their legs to receive the cup from the person behind them. Once back at the front, the cycle begins again: scooping water, passing back, pouring, and returning.

Give the teams a time limit of 30 seconds, or whatever makes sense for your group.

At the end of the time limit, the team with the most water in their end bucket wins!

You can shuffle up the teams or have plain ol' rematches—keep playing until everyone has cooled off or you run out of water!

SPONGE TOSS

AGES - ANY
GROUP SIZE - 6 OR MORE
TIME - 10 MINUTES
MATERIALS - BUCKETS, SPONGES, AND WATER

Like "Bucket Race," "Sponge Toss" is a wacky way to shed some heat, both thermal and competitive.

Divide the group into two teams and set a time limit—one minute is a good baseline.

The setup is similar to "Bucket Race"; there should be a full bucket of water for each team on one side of the playing field and an empty bucket for each team on the other side.

Half of each team should be on the end with the full buckets, and the other half of each team should be on the end with the empty buckets.

Players can use a sponge to soak up water from the full bucket, and then toss the sponge to their teammate near the empty bucket, who wrings out any remaining water into the bucket before tossing the sponge back.

Have players rotate on their sides so that no one person is doing all of the soaking, tossing, or wringing.

The game ends when time runs out—whichever team has the most water in their end bucket wins!

Reset and play again! Have folks switch roles or teams. No one wants to consistently be on the receiving end of a bunch of wet sponges!

BUCKET TOSS

AGES – ANY
GROUP SIZE – 6 OR MORE
TIME – 10 MINUTES
MATERIALS – BUCKETS, CUPS, AND WATER

"Bucket Toss" serves as one "final" water game, though, like with tag, there are certainly more variations that you could invent.

Divide players into two teams, and have the teams separate so that half of a team is on one side of a playing field and the other half is on the opposite side.

Set a time limit of a minute or two, during which the teams are trying to get as much water in the end bucket as possible.

One side of the field should have a full bucket of water, and the other side of the field an empty one.

Players on the full side are using a cup to scoop water from the bucket. They can then "toss" the water to the other side, where teammates are holding the bucket to "catch" the liquid. The cup should not be thrown, just the liquid within.

After each throw, players should rotate on their side to give everyone a chance to either throw or catch.

At the end of the time limit, the team with the most water in their bucket wins, though perhaps the team with the most water on their bodies is the real winner?

Reset and play again and again, all summer long!

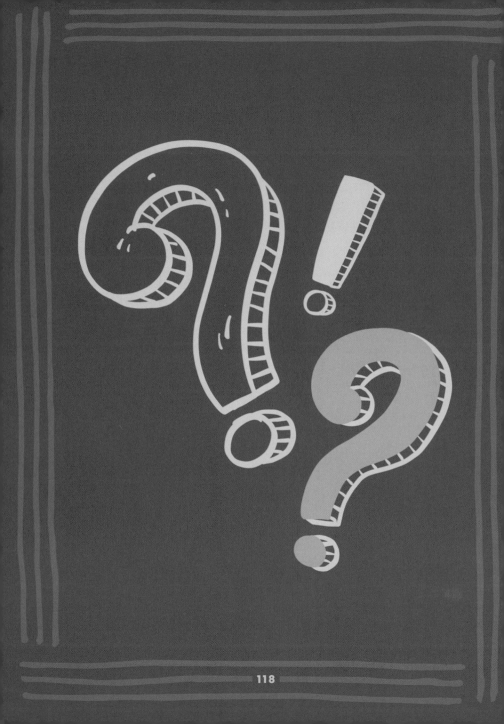

RIDDLES AND WORD GAMES

A little something to help pass the time—good for car rides or small moments between activities.

CUPCAKE

This word game goes like this: "If I have a cupcake, and I give it to Sally, who gives it to Bill, who gives it to Jeff, who has the cupcake?"

Whoever speaks first after you say "cupcake" for the last time "has" the cupcake.

For example, if you say the above line, and Skyler speaks first, she has the cupcake.

If you say, "If I have the cupcake, and I give it to my dog, who eats the cupcake entirely, who has the cupcake now?" *you* have the cupcake, because you are the first person to speak after saying "cupcake" for the last time when you said "now."

Encourage your players to try to discover the pattern, but make sure that they don't blurt out the explanation to everyone, so that they all get a chance to solve the puzzle. Players can demonstrate understanding by answering correctly, or, if they must, by whispering the solution to you.

Be creative—kids love outlandish paths for the cupcake to take!

BLACK MAGIC

This riddle requires two people to be in the know about the solution. It's a fun way to gain clout and add some mystery for the kids, especially if you and a coleader can be the ones running the riddle.

Have your coleader leave the area to a place where they definitely cannot hear you communicate with the group.

With the group, decide on an object that your partner will be trying to guess. Once you've decided, invite them back to the group.

Now, you should point out objects, asking your partner if that is "the one."

You will signal your partner that the true object is about to come up by pointing out a black object and asking if that's the one. Your partner should interpret this to mean that the next object you point to will be the one.

Stupify your players by consistently being able to communicate the mystery object to your partner "telepathically."

Following the same principles as "Cupcake," allow players the chance to try to solve the riddle.

PENGUINS

Present the following riddle aloud to your group:

"Two penguins are paddling a canoe through the desert. The one in the front says to the one in the back, 'Wears the paddle?' The one in the back says, 'Sure does!'—what are they talking about?"

Solution: The sand of the desert is *wearing* down the paddle blades.

You can allow players to ask "yes" or "no" questions as much as you can stand to answer them.

CHIMNEY

Present the following riddle aloud to your group:

"What can go up a chimney down, but not down a chimney up?"

Solution: An umbrella.

You can allow players to ask "yes" or "no" questions as much as you can stand to answer them.

TIPS ON "CASTING" SPECIAL ROLES AND SETTLING TIES

It may come as no surprise that kids love having a special role in a game. To reduce drama over being chosen, you can communicate that multiple players will get the chance to do the job. If that isn't enough, random trivia questions add a sense of merit-based decision-making that can put players at ease. Another rule that can work well is "if you ask to be _____, the answer is 'no,'" to avoid having players pile on the requests.

MOO OFF

A "Moo Off" is one way to settle a tie—have players stand toe to toe and simultaneously give their best impression of a cow. The winner can be the person with the longest moo, loudest moo, or most convincing moo. You, or the other players, are the judge!

SPLAT OFF

A "Splat Off" is another way to settle a tie. It connects naturally with the game "Splat!" (see page 62), but it can be used any time! Have players begin by standing back-to-back and announcing a trigger word, such as "coriander." Each time you say a word that is not "coriander," players should take another step away from each other. When you do say "coriander," it is a race to turn around, point, and be the first person to say "splat!" Whoever does this wins the tiebreaker.

Be creative! There are lots of ways to determine an ultimate champion, or you can always have kids share the title.

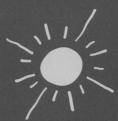

Emily Philpott has been working outside for nearly a decade, and playing outside for much longer than that. From a childhood creating imaginary worlds of dragons and mermaids and fairies with her sisters in the woods behind their home to a career as an outdoor adventure professional, Emily has always found a way to keep fun in her life. She is grateful for mentors and friends like the folks at Virginia Commonwealth University's Outdoor Adventure Program, Blue Sky Fund, Riverside Outfitters, and the Philadelphia Outward Bound School. Though she may have been able to game without them, the play certainly wouldn't have been so sweet.

ABOUT CIDER MILL PRESS BOOK PUBLISHERS

Good ideas ripen with time. From seed
to harvest, Cider Mill Press brings fine reading,
information, and entertainment together between
the covers of its creatively crafted books. Our
Cider Mill bears fruit twice a year, publishing
a new crop of titles each spring and fall.

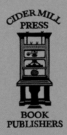

"Where Good Books Are Ready for Press"
501 Nelson Place
Nashville, Tennessee 37214

cidermillpress.com